MW01027861

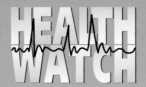

Sickle Cell Disease

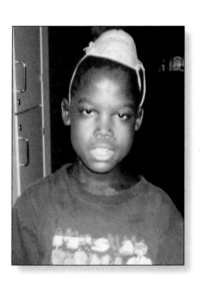

Susan Dudley Gold

Expert Review by Lillian McMahon, M.D.

Enslow Publishers, Inc.

40 Industrial Road	PO Box 38
Box 398	Aldershot
Berkeley Heights, NJ 07922	Hants GU12 6BP
USA	UK

http://www.enslow.com

Dedicated to Jeanne Vestal, who taught me so much about writing, about the children's book industry, and about enjoying life.

Acknowledgments
With thanks to:
Keone and Leslie Penn for their willingness to share their story.
Lillian McMahon, M.D., director, Boston Comprehensive Sickle Cell Center, and Associate Professor of Pediatrics and Medicine, Boston University School of Medicine, for her expert advice and review of this book.
My husband, John Gold, for his help and invaluable counsel in preparing this book.

Library of Congress Cataloging-in-Publication Data
Gold, Susan Dudley.
   Sickle cell disease / Susan Dudley Gold.
      p. cm. —— (Health watch)
Includes bibliographical references and index.
   ISBN 0-7660-1662-5 (hardcover)
   1. Sickle cell disease—Juvenile literature. [1. Sickle cell disease.
2. Diseases.] [DNLM: 1. Sickle Cell Disease—Popular Works.
WH 170 G18s 2001] I. Title. II. Health watch (Berkeley Heights, N.J.)
   RC641.7.S5 G64 2001
   616.1'527—dc21

                           00-012883

10 9 8 7 6 5 4 3 2 1

To Our Readers:
All Internet Addresses in this book were active and appropriate when we went to press. Any comments or suggestions can be sent by e-mail to Comments@enslow.com or to the address on the back cover.

Illustration and Photo Credits
Courtesy, Leslie Penn: pp. 1, 4, 6, 37, 38; © Susan Gold: p. 9; © PhotoDisc: pp. 10, 22, 25; © Jill Gregory: p. 12; © 1994 Corel Corp.: p. 16; courtesy North American Precis Syndicate, Inc.: p. 20; © Phil Skinner/*Atlanta Journal-Constitution*: p. 32.

Cover Illustrations
Large photo, courtesy, Leslie Penn; top inset, © Susan Gold; bottom inset, © PhotoDisc.

Contents

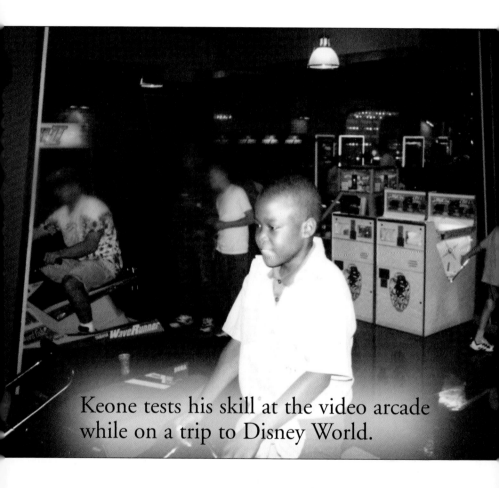

Keone tests his skill at the video arcade while on a trip to Disney World.

Chapter 1

Keone's Story

As a toddler, Keone Penn often got infections. He had pneumonia twice and so many fevers that his mother stopped counting the episodes. When he was five, the little boy had a **stroke**. Keone had to learn how to walk and talk all over again.

Leslie Penn, Keone's mother, recalls how her son screamed in pain. She cried herself when she saw him doubled over, barely able to breathe because of the painful attack that struck his body without warning.

"It would hurt so much, I wouldn't even want to blink," Keone told a reporter for the *Atlanta Journal-Constitution*. The year he turned twelve he went to the hospital eight times with fever, pain, and infections.

Keone's problems were caused by a condition called **sickle cell disease**, an inherited blood disorder that interferes with the flow of red blood cells through the body. It is most common in people with African backgrounds, but it can occur less often in those of other ethnic origins as well. Sickle cell disease blocks circulation and can cause

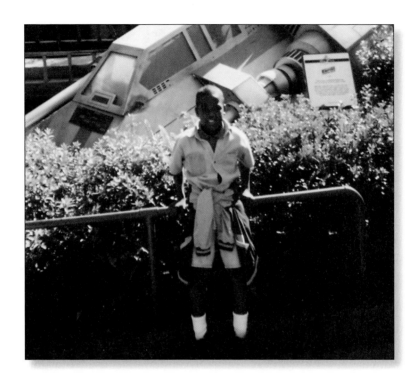

Keone, twelve, takes a break while visiting Disney World in Florida in November 1998 just before his transplant procedure was performed. The Make-A-Wish Foundation sponsored the trip to Disney.

people to be less resistant to certain infections. It can also cause kidney failure, seizures, strokes, and sometimes death. Sickle cell disease used to be incurable. People with severe forms of the disease often died young. Many did not live beyond their fifth birthday.

Ms. Penn first learned Keone had the disease when she took him to a doctor for a checkup when he was six months old. The doctor checked the results of a blood test done when Keone was born. The test showed that Keone had sickle cell disease. A long, hard road lay ahead:

monthly blood transfusions, infections, pain, stroke. But, finally, researchers had good news that neither Keone's mother nor his doctor ever expected: Keone had a chance for a cure.

Today new treatments and better medical care have extended the lives of many with the disease. Even more encouraging, some people—including Keone—have been cured.

In 1998, when Keone was twelve years old, he became the first person to receive transplanted **stem cells** to cure sickle cell disease. The cells were donated by a New York mother and her baby. The stem cells had been collected from blood in the mother's **placenta**—an organ that helps to nourish a developing baby—and from the baby's **umbilical cord**. Stem cells are cells that are formed early in the development of the baby and can be used to grow blood cells or other types of cells. In Keone's case, the cells were used to produce a new blood system and **bone marrow**. The new bone marrow produced healthy red blood cells that did not have a sickle shape. Two years after the procedure, doctors proclaimed Keone cured.

Chapter 2

What Is Sickle Cell Disease?

Keone Penn is one of two hundred fifty thousand children worldwide who develop sickle cell disease every year. The disease is actually a group of disorders that affect the red blood cells. Red blood cells serve as the body's oxygen delivery service. **Hemoglobin**, a **protein** inside the red blood cells, carries oxygen from the lungs to all parts of the body. Blood vessels and smaller **capillaries** provide the road system through which the blood cells travel.

Healthy red blood cells are round and pass easily through the vessels with their vital cargo of oxygen. But in people with sickle cell disease, the red blood cells become misshapen after they deliver oxygen to the organs. They form hard, sticky shapes that look like the crescent-shaped tools, called sickles, that are used to cut wheat. When these sickle-shaped cells try to pass through the blood vessels, they stick to the sides and interfere with

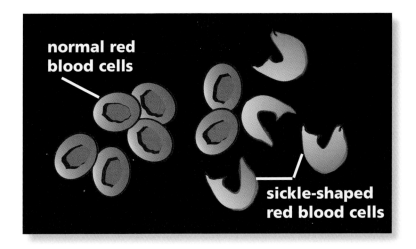

normal red
blood cells

sickle-shaped
red blood cells

*An illustration of normal human red blood cells is
pictured on left. Red blood cells from a person with
sickle cell disease are illustrated on right.*

the flow of blood. This slows the blood flow and reduces
the amount of oxygen that gets through to the rest of the
body. Sometimes the cells pile up and completely block
the way.

Those areas that receive no oxygen become painful and
inflamed. When the pain becomes extreme, the person
experiences what is called a **pain crisis**. If the blood is
blocked too long, it can damage organs and other parts of
the body. People with sickle cell disease have **anemia**, a
condition caused when there are too few red blood cells.
Anemia can make a person feel weak and tired.

Genes Are to Blame

Proteins are the body's work force. They are formed from
amino acids, molecules that link together to form a complex chain.

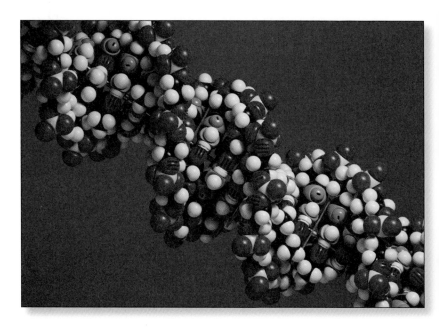

A model shows the strands of nucleotides that make up deoxyribonucleic acid (DNA).

Hair, fingernails, tendons, skin, and many other parts of the body are made of proteins. Proteins regulate what goes into and comes out of each cell. They also determine how the body moves, breathes, and gets oxygen. Proteins have thousands of jobs to do.

The instructions for making proteins come from **genes**, the "blueprint" that determines each person's traits. Every baby is born with a set of genes from the mother and a set of genes from the father. Genes direct whether a child will have curly or straight hair, big or small feet, and light or dark skin and eyes.

Genes are composed of tiny molecules of **deoxyribonucleic acid (DNA)**. Each DNA molecule is made up of long strands of material called **nucleotides**. Every portion of the strand appears in a certain order. This sequence signals the order in which amino acids are arranged in proteins. Two proteins can contain exactly the same amino acids but behave very differently, depending on how the amino acids are arranged. A change in only one amino acid can alter the way a protein acts in the body.

Sickle cell disease is an inherited condition, passed to a child through the parents' genes. Due to changes that occurred long ago, some of our ancestors' genes became faulty. Those faulty genes, passed down from one generation to the next, carry the wrong instructions to the body.

In the case of sickle cell disease, just one amino acid is substituted for another in hemoglobin, the protein found in red blood cells. This causes the hemoglobin to form long rods after it releases oxygen to the body. This, in turn, makes the red blood cells become sickle-shaped.

The genes people inherit from their parents determine the type of hemoglobin they will have. Many will have normal (AA) hemoglobin. Others will have one of the more than seven hundred abnormal types of hemoglobin, including those that lead to sickle cell disease. Only people who inherit two abnormal genes—one from their mother and one from their father—will have sickle cell disease.

People who inherit one sickle cell gene and one normal gene are said to have **sickle cell trait**. They do not develop the disease, but they can pass the gene along to their children.

Both Keone's mother and father have sickle cell trait. He has four half-sisters and half-brothers. None of them has the disease.

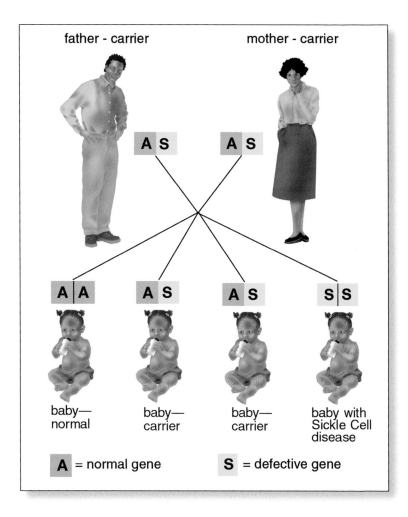

A baby must inherit two sickle cell genes to have sickle cell disease.

Surprisingly, people with sickle cell trait have an advantage over other people who do not have the trait. They are immune to a certain kind of **malaria**, a tropical blood disease spread by mosquitoes that is often fatal. Scientists believe that is one reason the faulty sickle cell gene spread in tropical regions. Those who had the gene survived malaria outbreaks and had children, many of whom also carried the gene.

A parent with a sickle cell gene has a 50 percent chance of passing the gene to his or her children. If both parents have sickle cell trait, their children have a 50 percent chance of inheriting sickle cell trait, a 25 percent chance of having sickle cell disease, and a 25 percent chance of inheriting normal red blood cell genes.

Scientists first discovered sickle cell disease in people who lived in West Africa or whose ancestors had come from that region. The disease is also found among people from other ethnic origins. It is fairly common in areas of Africa that lie along the equator, in parts of southern Italy, southern Greece, central India, Saudi Arabia, and Turkey.

Sickle cell disease is the most common inherited blood disease in the world. It affects millions of people. Doctors estimate that as many as one million people in Nigeria have the disease. About 30 percent of the people who live in some villages in India and 20 to 30 percent of those in some communities in southern Greece have inherited the sickle cell gene.

In the United States, about eighty thousand Americans have the disease. About seventy thousand of those are African Americans. One in ten African Americans has sickle cell trait.

Types of Sickle Cell Disease

There are several types of sickle cell disease in the United States. The three most common types are hemoglobin SS or **sickle cell anemia, hemoglobin SC disease**, and

sickle beta-thalassemia. Of the three, sickle cell anemia, the kind that Keone Penn had, is the most common. People with this form of the disease inherit the hemoglobin S (HbS) gene from both parents. The next most common and usually milder type is hemoglobin SC disease. Those with this type inherit one HbS gene and one hemoglobin C (HbC) gene. Sickle beta-thalassemia is less common and may be more severe. It occurs when a person inherits an HbS gene and a gene for beta-thalassemia. **Thalassemia** is a type of anemia that prevents a person from producing enough hemoglobin.

Chapter 3

Symptoms

Babies with sickle cell disease don't usually have any **symptoms** of the disease until they are about six months old. Then, without warning, the baby's hands and feet may swell, and he or she may scream in pain.

"He started crying and crying, and he wouldn't stop," said the mother of a young boy whose symptoms began when he was one year old. Seye Arise, whose story was featured in a *Time* magazine article, had a stroke when he was four years old. This caused him to limp.

A stroke occurs when the brain does not receive the amount of oxygen it needs to function normally.

Some people have a form of sickle cell disease that is so mild it may never be diagnosed. They may have few symptoms and live a normal life span. Others, with harsher forms of the disease, may have painful joints, swollen arms and legs, and problems with vision.

The worst cases damage the brain, lungs, or other organs and can result in death. **Acute chest syndrome**, a

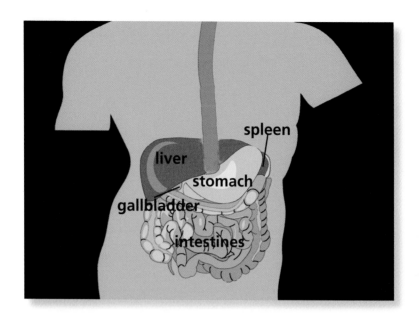

The spleen helps fight off infection. The person's left side is pictured on the right in the illustration.

condition that results in chest pain, fast breathing, and coughing, is a major cause of death in these cases.

About 8 percent of those with the disease have a stroke by the time they reach fourteen. They are much less likely to have stroke after that age. Another problem for those with sickle cell disease, especially children, is infection. The **spleen**, located in the left side of the abdomen, helps the body fight off infection. During the first few years of a baby's life, the spleen helps the body to fight many different types of **bacteria**, germs that invade the body and can cause it harm. This protects the person from certain bacteria throughout life.

The spleen also filters the red and white blood cells. During this filtering process, red blood cells affected by sickle cell disease clog the spleen and destroy it. By the time a child is one or two, the spleen is no longer able to protect against germs. For the first five years of their lives, children with sickle cell disease have to take **antibiotics**— medicines that fight germs—to prevent infection. Without such medicines, these children might die from infectious diseases such as pneumonia.

Hand-foot syndrome is another symptom that strikes young children with sickle cell. The small bones in the hands and feet become painful. About half of those with the disease develop hand-foot syndrome by the age of two. It is rare in children older than five.

Children with sickle cell disease may grow more slowly or be smaller than other children their age. Blood cells normally last 120 days. Sickle cells may survive only ten to twelve days. That means the bone marrow, where red blood cells are made, has to work harder and faster to keep the body supplied with the needed blood cells. The energy and protein that would normally help a child grow are instead being used to create red blood cells. The products from all the dying red blood cells can cause **jaundice**, a condition related to the liver that causes the skin and eyes to have a yellowish color.

People with this disease also suffer from gallstones, a painful condition that affects the gallbladder. In one study, 40 percent of the sickle cell patients had gallstones by the time they were twenty.

People with the disease may have severe bone pain. Areas that are painful include the knees, elbows, shoulders, ribs, spine, and pelvis. Leg ulcers are a major problem for some adults.

Women with sickle cell disease may develop health problems if they become pregnant. They are more likely to have miscarriages or give birth to underweight babies than other mothers.

Other symptoms of the disease include kidney failure, eye damage, and brain damage from stroke.

Because of the number of deaths early in the disease, the average life span for males in the United States with sickle cell disease is forty-two. Females with the disease live an average of forty-eight years. But some people live much longer. Those with mild forms live almost as long as those who do not have the disease.

Keone's Symptoms

Between the ages of one and three, Keone had infections and fevers constantly. Serious infections sent him to the hospital, where nurses gave him antibiotics to fight germs. The medical staff inserted a needle into his vein and the antibiotics flowed into his bloodstream. This is called an **intravenous injection**, or **IV**. Keone usually had to stay at the hospital for ten days at a time. "We were in the hospital quite a bit in those early years," said his mother.

At age three, Keone began to respond to the antibiotics he had to take every day. For a couple of years, the toddler developed like any other child. He quickly learned the alphabet. In kindergarten, he recited numbers and was an eager learner. Then one day, when he was five, his teacher called home to tell Keone's mother that he had behaved strangely that day. When the teacher had asked him to pick up a paper and deposit it in the trash bin, he had thrown it on the floor instead. He seemed unaware of what was happening around him.

Worried, Leslie Penn watched as Keone stepped off the school bus. She noted that his mouth had twisted into an odd shape. He couldn't answer simple questions when she asked him what his name was or where he lived. At the hospital, doctors at first thought he might have a brain tumor. But after tests, they concluded Keone had had a stroke.

A procedure called a blood exchange provided Keone with fresh red blood cells. The hospital staff injected a needle in one arm and drained some of Keone's blood. At the same time, they injected another needle in the other arm and pumped healthy new blood into his body. The healthy blood carried needed oxygen to Keone's organs.

The stroke left Keone unable to walk or talk. He could not move his right side at all. After the stroke, Keone no longer knew his ABCs. Counting to ten was too difficult for him.

Doctors predicted that the five-year-old would have to spend the rest of his life in a nursing home. But Keone and his mother didn't give up. Keone spent hours work- ing with a physical therapist doing exercises to strengthen his muscles. A speech therapist taught him how to speak again. Slowly, he recovered.

"Keone has had several miracles in his life," his mother said. "This was one of them. He came all the way back."

To look at Keone after his recovery, no one would have known he had had a stroke. He could walk and talk normally. The only lasting effect from the stroke is a

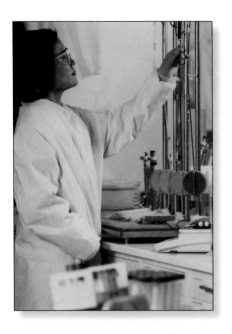

A technician prepares blood for a transfusion.

learning disability, which makes it harder for Keone to reason. Because of the learning disability, Keone does not do well in large groups.

After the stroke, Keone began receiving blood transfusions every week. The medical staff inserted a needle into his vein. Blood from a donor traveled through a tube into the needle and through Keone's veins. For a while, the new healthy blood replaced the sickle-shaped blood. But soon new sickle-shaped blood cells formed in Keone's bone marrow and replaced the healthy blood cells. Later Keone had transfusions every two weeks, then once a month.

A new transfusion of blood made Keone feel stronger. The yellow in his eyes, caused by jaundice, disappeared. He had more energy. Then as sickled blood cells gradually replaced healthy ones, Keone became weaker and more tired. He developed jaundice.

"You could tell when he needed a transfusion," his mother said, "because his eyes turned yellow."

Then the cycle would begin anew with a fresh transfusion of healthy blood.

Chapter 4

Diagnosis and Treatment

C hildren with sickle cell disease used to be more likely to die during their first year of life than at any other time. Because people usually don't have symptoms of sickle cell disease until they reach the age of one, doctors were often unaware that babies had the disease. Now many of the deaths are prevented because blood tests can identify babies who have the disease, and they can be treated early.

Before becoming parents, people who think they may have sickle cell trait can have a blood test to see if they carry the sickle cell gene. If both people carry the gene, they may decide not to have children. If they decide to have a child, there is a 25 percent chance that the child will be born with sickle cell disease. Because the disease is so common worldwide, many doctors urge everyone to have the blood test before deciding to become parents.

Modern technology has made it possible for doctors to

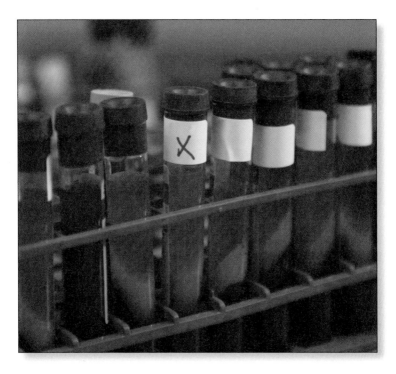

Test tubes hold blood ready to be tested. A blood test done at birth can determine whether a baby has sickle cell disease.

test unborn babies for sickle cell disease. During the mother's pregnancy, the doctor uses a long needle to extract fluid from around the developing baby. This test is called **amniocentesis**. Technicians then study the genes in the fluid to see if there are any sickle cell genes. If two sickle cell genes are present, that means the baby will be born with sickle cell disease. A similar test can be done on tissue collected with a needle from the outer membrane of the placenta.

Most hospitals in the United States test all babies for sickle cell disease as soon as they are born. The blood test shows whether babies have the disease or sickle cell trait.

Keone was given this test at birth, but for some unknown reason his mother wasn't told of the results until he was six months old.

Another sign of the disease is hand-foot syndrome. If a child has the syndrome, it is likely that he or she has sickle cell disease.

Treating Sickle Cell Disease

Until a short while ago, doctors could only treat the symptoms of sickle cell disease. There was no cure. Today, new kinds of treatments have cured Keone Penn and several other people of the disease. But Keone and others continue to have health problems brought on by the treatment. Researchers hope that someday soon such experimental treatments will be able to cure many people with sickle cell disease safely and effectively.

Because the treatment that cured Keone is so risky, it is better to continue to treat the symptoms of those with mild to moderate sickle cell disease rather than try to cure them. Doctors have many ways to treat the disease that can make it much easier to live with.

Soon after a baby is born with sickle cell disease, it is important to protect him or her from germs. It matters because the spleen, which normally helps fight off infection, often does not work properly in people with sickle cell disease. In addition to the routine vaccines given to fight off mumps, measles, and other childhood diseases, doctors give babies with sickle cell disease a vaccine against pneumonia. Some children must take antibiotics twice a day to fight off infections. Doctors also give patients medicines to ease the pain from sickle cell disease and vitamins to supplement their diet. Children with sickle cell disease take folic acid, a vitamin that helps build their red blood cells.

From the time they are born until they are five years old, children with sickle cell disease take penicillin twice a day or receive monthly shots of long-acting penicillin. This medicine kills bacteria that used to cause many deaths among small children with the disease.

Because sickle cell disease can cause vision problems, a yearly eye exam is important for people with the disease.

Doctors use Doppler **ultrasound** machinery to learn if people with the disease are likely to have a stroke. The equipment, named after Austrian scientist Christian Johann Doppler, uses sound waves to record an image of the blood circulating inside a person's blood vessels. The sound waves bounce off certain parts that are thicker than the surrounding area. This creates a picture doctors can use to see whether the person's blood vessels are becoming blocked and predicts which children are most likely to develop a stroke.

Another machine—a **magnetic resonance imaging (MRI) scanner**—can also be used to check children for brain damage. In an MRI, magnetic rays scan the brain. A computer shows the structures inside the head and helps identify any damage done. Doctors can then give treatments such as monthly blood transfusions to prevent further damage.

People with severe sickle cell disease may get regular transfusions of blood, as Keone did. The round, healthy blood cells flow easily through the body, delivering

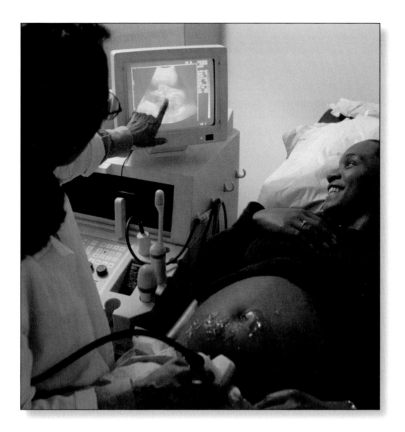

A technician uses an ultrasound machine to check on a developing baby in the mother's womb. The equipment can also be used to detect signs of a stroke.

needed oxygen. The treatment is only temporary, however. New sickle-shaped blood cells continue to form in the bone marrow. In a month or less, people with the disease may need another transfusion.

The treatment also has a bad side effect. Because they are constantly receiving new red blood cells that are rich in iron, people with sickle cell disease can accumulate too much of the metal. Iron helps form hemoglobin and plays a key role in delivering needed oxygen to cells. Like any heavy metal, though, iron in large quantities can cause serious damage to a person's lungs, brain, liver, and heart.

People with sickle cell disease must always be on the alert for infections. Because the disease reduces the body's ability to fight off germs, infections can develop rapidly. Such infections are serious and can sometimes be fatal if they are not treated quickly. When fever develops, a person with sickle cell disease needs medical attention right away. The person receives fluids through an IV to prevent **dehydration** and antibiotics to fight the infection. The patient may also receive pain medication. After several days of treatment, the patient may be able to go home. But sometimes patients must spend a week or longer in the hospital for treatment. Keone usually had to stay ten days each time he went to the hospital. It took that long for the antibiotics to work.

Doctors tell people with sickle cell disease to drink plenty of fluids, stay rested, and avoid crowds where people may be spreading cold or flu germs. People with the disease should try to stay warm in winter and cool in summer.

New Treatments

In the 1990s, doctors made remarkable breakthroughs in curing and treating sickle cell disease. Scientists found two ways of curing the disease. A bone marrow transplant was the first treatment to cure a sickle cell patient successfully. The second treatment, stem cell transplant, is the one that cured Keone. Both methods are experimental and risky. Experimental treatments have not been used long enough for doctors to know for sure that they work or what the side effects may be. But initial studies show that these treatments may help at least some of the people with the disease or disorder. More than one hundred children have been cured using one technique or the other.

In the first method, healthy bone marrow is transplanted from a sister or brother whose genes closely match those of the patient. The technique was first used in patients with leukemia.

In both techniques, patients take strong drugs that poison the body and kill all the bone marrow. Treatment with these drugs, called **chemotherapy**, may cause patients to lose their hair. Many also feel nauseous and don't want to eat anything. They become weak and tired. The procedure is risky because the bone marrow makes white blood cells that fight off disease and infection. Without it, germs from a cold or the flu can take over the body. Infections and other causes kill from 5 percent to 8 percent of children with blood diseases who have bone marrow transplants.

Once the bone marrow is dead, doctors inject the healthy bone marrow from a brother or sister into the patient. The new bone marrow grows white blood cells and healthy red blood cells that do not form sickle shapes. Medical staff watch patients closely during this time. Patients take heavy doses of antibiotics to guard against infections until the new white blood cells grow. Other medicines called corticosteroids reduce inflammation and swelling.

Some patients get **graft-versus-host disease** (GVHD). The body's white blood cells guard against germs and other harmful agents by attacking foreign substances. If the new bone marrow (the "graft") identifies the body (the "host") as foreign, the white blood cells will attack the body's organs. This makes patients very sick. They will vomit and have stomach cramps and diarrhea. Patients must take powerful drugs that suppress the immune system and keep the transplanted cells from fighting the patient's body. This keeps the white blood cells under control until the new cells "get used to" their new surroundings.

These powerful drugs can save people's lives. But they, too, can cause problems. When taken for a long time, steroids can cause stomach ulcers and upsets, thin bones, high blood pressure, depression, weight gain, and vision problems. They can also interfere with a child's growth. For these reasons, doctors try to limit the amount of steroids patients use over a long period of time. Immune suppressant drugs help control graft-versus-host disease, but they interfere with the body's defense against germs.

Despite these problems, those who receive transplants from sisters and brothers have a very good chance of being cured of sickle cell disease. About 90 percent of those receiving bone marrow from brothers or sisters have no further signs of sickle cell disease after their transplant procedure.

Chapter 5

Keone's Cure

After his stroke, Keone's life became a battle against sickle cell disease. He caught chicken pox three times because his immune system wasn't working properly. Every month Keone had to have a blood transfusion. Each time he had an infection, he had to spend ten days in the hospital. There, antibiotics dripped into his veins through an IV needle. He missed so much school that a tutor taught him at home and in the hospital.

The many injections scarred Keone's veins. During an operation, doctors installed a device in Keone's chest called a **Portacath**. A Portacath is one of two types of central venous catheter, or C-line, that make it easier to deliver blood and medicines to patients. Blood transfusions or antibiotics are injected into the Portacath, which feeds the liquids into the bloodstream. This meant Keone no longer had to have a needle inserted in his arm for each treatment.

The frequent blood transfusions made the level of iron

in Keone's blood skyrocket. The transfusions boosted his iron levels from a normal count of 500 mg/100 ml to well over 5,000 mg/100 ml. At one point, Keone's iron counts were so high that the disbelieving doctor ordered them retested.

Keone received shots just under the skin to remove the high amounts of iron. But infections plagued him, and he didn't do well. He had more and more painful episodes. The pain usually affected his back. "He'd be screaming in pain," said his mother. "It was so bad he would double over."

Leslie Penn recalled one afternoon Keone went to the mall with his cousins. It was the day after Thanksgiving in 1998, when Keone was twelve years old. His muscles became so tight he couldn't walk. His cousins had to carry him home.

"It got to the point where the disease was out of control," his mother said. "Nothing seemed to be working." Doctors told her that Keone might not live more than five more years. The bone marrow transplants that had cured some children would not help Keone. He had half-brothers and half-sisters but no full brother or sister who could donate bone marrow.

A Chance for a Cure

Researchers at Egleston Children's Hospital (now known as Children's Healthcare of Atlanta at Egleston) had been experimenting with stem cell transplants. They collected stem cells from mothers' placentas and babies' umbilical cords. The researchers then used the stem cells to grow bone marrow. The person receiving the transplant didn't have to be related to the people donating the stem cells. The procedure had worked on a few patients with leukemia. It had never been tried on a sickle cell patient before.

Doctors asked Keone and his mother if he would like to be the first person with sickle cell disease to try the experimental treatment. He would have to endure chemotherapy and take powerful medicines for months. If things went wrong, dangerous infections could kill Keone. The doctors said Keone had a 50-50 chance of being cured. Keone and his mother believed they had little choice. The disease was becoming worse. Here, at least, was a chance to be well.

"I don't want to die," Keone told a reporter before the transplant, "but I don't want to live like this, either."

In early December 1998, Keone began chemotherapy to kill his bone marrow. The first week he did fine. By the second week, however, he began to feel the effects of the powerful medicines. "He would grab handfuls of hair and pull it out to gross out his mama," said Keone's mother.

On December 11, doctors injected the stem cells into Keone's bloodstream. "It was a little IV bag with pink stuff in it," recalled his mother. "It ran through in four minutes. It was a real anticlimax." Keone gave the needle a last push to inject the final cells into his bloodstream. The stem cells lodged inside his bones, where Keone's marrow had been. They began forming new bone marrow, which would produce new blood cells for Keone. The treatment cost about $200,000, paid for by his mother's health insurance.

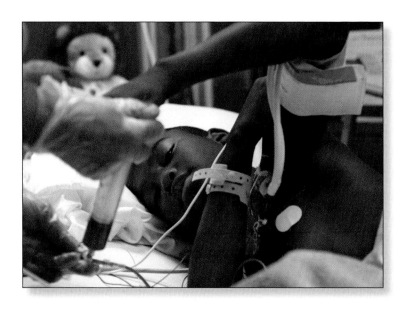

Keone helps push the last portion of donated stem cells into the tube that will carry it into his system.

Weak from the chemotherapy, Keone spent much of the next few weeks sleeping. Christmas that year wasn't much fun. Gifts from friendly strangers and family covered his hospital bed, but Keone was too weak and sick to open them. He didn't feel like eating the Christmas dinner his aunt brought to his room.

Visitors had to wear masks to avoid spreading germs. The room had special equipment to draw out germs and bacteria. In honor of its young occupant, the staff nicknamed Keone's room "Penn Palace 361." He would live there for two months.

Medical staff tested Keone's blood every day. The number of new blood cells steadily grew, a good sign. Then, during the first week in January, Keone had a seizure. A seizure occurs when the brain's electrical currents go out of control. Keone stopped breathing. Doctors thought he might die. They rushed him to a special area of the hospital where he received intensive care. Keone rallied, and in three days he returned to Penn Palace.

On January 16, 1999, Keone left the hospital. He wore a blue paper mask to keep out germs. Crowds were off-limits. But he was ecstatic to be going home.

Almost two years later, doctors have proclaimed Keone cured of sickle cell disease. His blood shows no signs of the sickle-shaped cells that once filled his veins. But the treatment and the effects of his medicines have taken a toll. In August 1999, Keone went back to school for the first time since his transplant. The eighth-grader lasted one day. Graft-versus-host disease—his mother calls it the "big, bad demon"—landed him in the hospital again. Keone still struggles with GVHD. Doctors hope it will disappear in a year or two.

Keone's joints are damaged, affected by the steroids he takes to reduce swelling and infection. Sickle cell may also have broken down the joints before he was cured of the disease. His doctors say Keone will eventually need replacements for both knees and both hips.

Keone is small for his age. At fourteen, he is only four feet nine inches tall. Steroids have slowed his growth. He is slowly cutting back on the medicine. When he first left the hospital, Keone had to swallow sixteen pills twice a day. Now he has a tube that connects to his stomach. Most of his medicine can be taken in liquid form through the tube, though he still has to swallow a few pills.

Back at school once again, Keone studies language arts

and math. He learns other subjects at home from a tutor. The GVHD makes him feel nauseous now and then. He has had to have IVs and food through a tube during those times when he couldn't eat. "As soon as we get over one hurdle," said his mother wearily, "there's another waiting for us."

Just recently, however, a hurdle brought good news. Keone caught a bad cold. He developed a cough, but he was able to fight off the cold without going to the hospital. His new immune system was strong enough to defeat the germs. "That was a really good sign," his mother said.

Other Experimental Treatments

Since Keone received the stem cell transplant, doctors have done the procedure on several other children. One, in Florida, is doing very well. But because of the risk and side effects of transplants, scientists continue to search for safer and simpler treatments and cures. Researchers are experimenting with nitric oxide, a colorless gas found in the body. The gas causes muscle cells in the blood vessels to relax. This enlarges the passageway in the vessels and allows more blood to flow through. Results from one study show that inhaling a small amount of the gas may increase the blood flow in people with sickle cell disease. The gas molecules attach themselves to the hemoglobin in the red blood cells and expand the blood vessels as they travel through. This increased blood flow may be one way to prevent pain crises and other problems caused by sickle cell.

Doctors are learning better ways of treating the disease.

Frequent blood transfusions and early medical care can reduce the effect of the disease on various organs. Such care has reduced the number of strokes in children with sickle cell. Doctors are using ultrasound to identify children at risk for stroke and MRI scans to check children for brain damage. Recent studies have shown that the disease may cause brain damage even in infants who have few symptoms. Those findings may prompt doctors to begin treatments such as blood transfusions at a much earlier age.

Other research focuses on fetal red blood cells—those found in the developing baby before birth. A medicine called **hydroxyurea** increases the fetal hemoglobin in red blood cells. The medicine has reduced the symptoms of sickle cell disease in some people. It is now being studied for use in children.

Red blood cells with fetal hemoglobin do not form the typical sickle shape. This is true even in **fetuses**—developing babies—that eventually have sickle cell disease. Researchers hope to learn the best way for people with sickle cell disease to increase their production of fetal hemoglobin and fetal cells. The answers to such questions may lead to therapies that prevent sickle-shaped red blood cells from forming in people with the disease.

Some scientists are exploring **gene therapy**, hoping to find a way to replace the genes that cause sickle cell disease with healthy genes.

Chapter 6

Living With Sickle Cell Disease

People with sickle cell disease are living longer today because of better medical care. Kerry Norwood learned he had the disease when he was three years old. Doctors at the time predicted he would die before he reached the age of seven.

His mother, Berrutha Harper, pushed doctors and medical staff to get him the best medical care possible. Through her efforts, Grady Memorial Hospital established the Georgia Comprehensive Sickle Cell Center at Grady Health System. The center focuses its efforts on caring for patients with sickle cell disease. Staff members also work to educate families about the disease.

Today, at thirty-three, Ms. Harper's son, Kerry, is married, holds a full-time job, and says he is "one of the healthiest sickle cell patients around," according to the *Atlanta Journal-Constitution*.

The worst sickle cell symptoms usually begin during

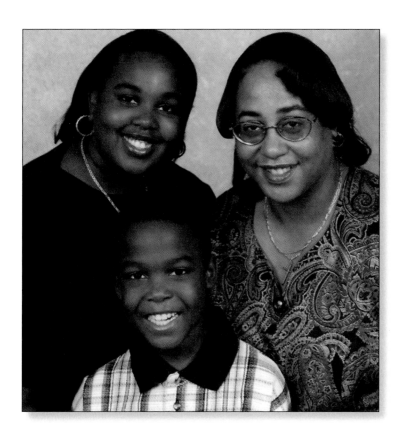

Keone, center, with his sister, Seterria Cuthrell, left, and his mother, Leslie Penn. The photo was taken around 1996 when Keone was ten years old.

childhood and early adulthood. Some patients are sicker when they are children while others suffer more as adults.

For Keone, living without sickle cell disease has been as much of a challenge as living with it. A teenager now, he dislikes anything that sets him apart from his friends. He refuses to use a cane, which he got when his knees began to bother him. He still struggles with GVHD. Some days he wonders if the cure was worth it.

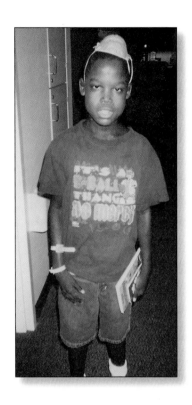

But other days he talks of his plans to become a chef and run his own restaurant. He goes to the movies with his buddy, David Greenburg, a medical student who volunteered to be Keone's friend. They eat out and have fun doing other activities together. Keone also spends time with his older cousin, who at sixteen is twice his size.

"We take one day at a time and keep hoping for better," his mother said. "I tell Keone that everyone has to deal with something. This is your slice of the pie."

Keone at the hospital after receiving the world's first stem cell transplant for sickle cell disease. The mask on top of his head helps block out germs.

Further Reading

Baldwin, Joyce. *DNA Pioneer: James Watson and the Double Helix*. New York: Walker & Company, 1994.

Balkwill, Fran. *DNA Is Here to Stay*. New York: The Lerner Publishing Group, 1993.

Ballard, Carol. *The Heart & Circulatory System* (The Human Body). Austin, Texas: Raintree/Steck Vaughn, 1997.

Beshore, George. *Sickle Cell Anemia* (A Venture Book). New York: Franklin Watts, 1994.

Bloom, Miriam. *Understanding Sickle Cell Disease* (Understanding Health and Sickness Series). Jackson, Miss.: University Press of Mississippi, 1995.

Edelson, Edward. *Genetics & Heredity*. Broomall, Penn.: Chelsea House, 1991.

Fridell, Ron. *DNA Fingerprinting: The Ultimate Identity*. New York: Franklin Watts, 2001.

Kelly, Pat. *Coping With Sickle-Cell Anemia*. New York: Rosen Publishing Group, 1999.

Kidd, J.S., and Renee A. Kidd. *Life Lines: The Story of the New Genetics*. New York: Facts on File, 1998.

Lampton, Christopher F. *DNA Fingerprinting*. New York: Franklin Watts, 1991.

Silverstein, Alvin, et al. *Sickle Cell Anemia* (Diseases and People). Berkeley Heights, N.J.: Enslow Publishers, Inc., 1997.

Tapper, Melbourne. *In the Blood: Sickle Cell Anemia & the Politics of Race* (Critical Histories). Philadelphia: University of Pennsylvania Press, 1999.

Walker, Dava. *Puzzles.* Lollipop Power, Inc., 1996.

Wilcox, Frank H. *DNA: The Threat of Life.* New York: The Lerner Publishing Group, 1988.

For More Information

The following is a list of organizations and Web sites that deal with sickle cell disease.

Organizations

Agency for Health Care Policy and Research
Publications Clearinghouse, P.O. Box 8547&127, Silver Spring, MD 20907, (800) 358-9295; <http://www.ahcpr.gov>

American Sickle Cell Anemia Association
10300 Carnegie Avenue, Cleveland Clinic/East Office Building (EEb18), Cleveland, OH 44106; (216) 229-8600; <http://www.ascaa.org>

Boston Comprehensive Sickle Cell Center
Boston Medical Center, One Boston Medical Center Place, FGH-2, Boston MA 02118, (617) 414-5727; Lillian McMahon, M.D., director, e-mail: lmcmahon@bu.edu

Center for Sickle Cell Disease
Howard University, 2121 Georgia Avenue, NW, Washington, D.C. 20059, (202) 806-7930; <http://www.huhosp.org/sicklecell/index.htm>

Cincinnati Comprehensive Sickle Cell Center
Children's Hospital Medical Center, 3333 Burnet Avenue, Cincinnati, OH 45229-3039, (800) 344-2462, (513) 559-4200; <http://www.cincinnatichildrens.org/programs_services/108/index.asp>

Comprehensive Sickle Cell Center—Medical College of Georgia

Medical College of Georgia, 1120 15th Street, FF-100 Augusta, GA 30912; (706) 721-2196; <http://www.usg.edu/admin/icapp/centers/medical/med_sickle.html>

Cooley's Anemia Foundation

Thalassemia Action Group, 129-09 26th Avenue #203, Flushing, NY 11354, (800) 522-7222, (718) 321-CURE (2873); <http://www.thalassemia.org>

Genetic Disease Resource Center

California State Department of Health Services, Genetic Disease Resource Center, 2151 Berkeley Way, Annex 4, Berkeley, CA 94704, (510) 540-2534

Georgia Comprehensive Sickle Cell Center

P.O. Box 109, Grady Memorial Hospital, 80 Butler Street, SE, Atlanta, GA 30303, (404) 616-3572; <http://www.emory.edu/PEDS/SICKLE>

March of Dimes Birth Defects Foundation

1275 Mamaroneck Avenue, White Plains, NY 10605, (800) 367-6630; <http://www.modimes.org>

National Center for Education in Maternal and Child Health

2000 15th Street, North, Suite 701, Arlington, VA 22201, (703) 524-7802; <http://www.ncemch.org>

National Heart, Lung, and Blood Institute

National Institutes of Health, Sickle Cell Disease Branch, Two Rockledge Centre, Room 10148, MSC 7950, Bethesda, MD 20892-7950, (301) 435-0055; <http://www.nhlbi.nih.gov/health/public/blood/index.htm>

National Maternal and Child Health Clearinghouse
8201 Greensboro Drive, Suite 600, McLean, VA
22102, (703) 821-8955

Sickle Cell Disease Association of America
200 Corporate Point, Suite 495, Culver City, CA
90230-7633, (800) 421-8453, (310) 216-6363;
<http://www.sicklecelldisease.org>

Internet Resources

<http://www.curtis1.com>
Site of Curtis R. Schneider, a California teacher; offers
information and Web site links to many areas of
human disease.

<http://sickle.bwh.harvard.edu>
Web site of Joint Center for Sickle Cell and
Thalassemic Disorders, joint program of Harvard
Medical School and Brigham and Women's Hospital

<http://wellweb.com/INDEX/QSICKLE.htm>
Wellness Web site with tips and resources from
conventional and alternative medicine

<http://www.thalassemia.org.cy>
Site of Thalassemia International Federation

Glossary

acute chest syndrome—A serious condition that causes the person to breathe rapidly, cough, and have chest pain. It is a major cause of death in sickle cell patients.

amino acids—Molecules that bond together to form proteins.

amniocentesis—A test of fetal cells using a needle to withdraw fluid surrounding the developing baby.

anemia—A condition in which a person has too few red blood cells. A person with anemia feels weak and tired.

antibiotics—Medicines used to combat germs and infection.

bacteria—Germs that invade the body and can cause it harm.

bone marrow—The soft material inside the bones where blood cells are made.

capillaries—Tiny blood vessels that run from the veins and arteries to all parts of the body.

chemotherapy—Drug treatment used to kill cells.

dehydration—A condition caused by an excessive loss of water from the body.

deoxyribonucleic acid (DNA)—Complex strands that make up the genetic material of living things.

fetus—A developing baby.

genes—The biological units that determine a person's traits. People inherit an equal number of genes from their mothers and their fathers.

gene therapy—Experimental treatment that replaces faulty genes with healthy ones.

graft-versus-host disease—A disorder caused when transplanted cells attack the body.

hand-foot syndrome—A painful condition of the hands and feet. Usually found in very young children.

hemoglobin—A protein molecule in red blood cells that carries oxygen from the lungs to other parts of the body.

hemoglobin SC disease—A common form of sickle cell disease. It results from inheriting two different sickle cell genes, hemoglobin S and hemoglobin C.

hydroxyurea—A medicine that increases the fetal hemoglobin in red blood cells; used to reduce the symptoms of sickle cell disease.

intravenous injection (IV)—Administering medication or other substances through a needle inserted in a person's vein.

jaundice—A condition that causes the skin to turn yellow.

magnetic resonance imaging (MRI) scanner—A device that uses magnetic rays to scan the brain.

malaria—A tropical blood disease spread by mosquitoes.

nucleotide—small units of molecules that join together to form DNA.

pain crisis—Severe pain caused when sickle-shaped blood cells clog blood vessels. This prevents the area from getting enough oxygen.

placenta—An organ that helps nourish a developing baby.

Portacath—A device surgically implanted in a person through which injections can be made.

protein—Long chains of amino acids that perform many tasks in the body.

sickle beta-thalassemia—A less common type of sickle cell disease. It derives from inheriting a hemoglobin S gene and a gene for b-thalassemia.

sickle cell anemia—The most common form of sickle cell disease. People with this disease inherit two hemoglobin S genes from their parents. Also known as hemoglobin SS disease.

sickle cell disease—A group of inherited blood disorders in which misshapen red blood cells interfere with the flow of blood through the body. It is the most common genetic blood disease in the world.

sickle cell trait—A condition in which a person inherits one sickle cell gene. The person will not have sickle cell disease but can pass on the sickle cell gene to his or her children.

spleen—The organ located in the left side of the abdomen responsible for fighting infection.

stem cells—Cells formed early in a baby's development that can be used to grow various types of cells.

stroke—A disorder caused when not enough oxygen reaches the brain. It can interfere with the ability to walk, talk, and think.

symptom—Signs of a disease or disorder.

thalassemia—A type of anemia that prevents a person from producing enough hemoglobin.

ultrasound—A technique using sound waves to record an image of the blood circulating inside the blood vessels.

umbilical cord—The flexible cord that connects the developing baby to the mother.

Index